COLOSTOMY DIET COOKBOOK FOR ALL

Healing Recipes: Delicious, Gut-Friendly Meals for Colostomy Patients

DR. D. JOHNSTON

COPYRIGHT © 2024 by [DR.D.JOHNSTON]

All rights reserved. No part of this publication may be reproduced, distributed, or transmitted in any form or by any means, including photocopying, recording, or other electronic or mechanical methods, without the prior written permission of the publisher, except in the case of brief quotations embodied in critical reviews and certain other noncommercial uses permitted by copyright law.

CONTENTS

INTRODUCTION ----------------------------------- 9

Chapter 1: ------------------------------------ 13

Welcome Message ---------------------------- 13

    The Purpose of This Cookbook ---------------- 13

    How to Use This Cookbook -------------------- 14

Chapter 2: ------------------------------------ 17

Understanding a Colostomy ------------------- 17

    Types of Colostomies ------------------------- 17

    Common Concerns After Colostomy Surgery ----- 18

    Myths About Colostomies --------------------- 19

Chapter 3: ------------------------------------ 21

Nutrition Basics ------------------------------ 21

    Importance of a Balanced Diet for Colostomy Patients -- 21

    Key Nutrients for Colostomy Patients ---------- 22

Chapter 4: ------------------------------------ 25

Colostomy Diet Principles --------------------- 25

    Foods to Avoid After Colostomy Surgery ---------- 25

    Foods to Include After Colostomy Surgery -------- 26

    Managing Gas and Odor ----------------------------- 28

    Hydration Tips -- 29

Chapter 5: -- 31

Special Considerations ---------------------------------- 31

    Managing Diarrhea After Colostomy Surgery ----- 31

    Managing Constipation After Colostomy Surgery 32

    Dealing with Blockages (Stoma Obstruction) ------ 33

Chapter 6: -- 35

Post-Surgery Diet Phases -------------------------------- 35

    Initial Post-Surgery Diet (First Few Weeks) ------- 35

    Transitioning to a Regular Diet (After a Few Weeks) --- 36

Chapter 7: -- 39

Meal Planning Tips -------------------------------------- 39

    Creating a Balanced Meal Plan After Colostomy Surgery -- 39

    Shopping List Essentials: ----------------------------- 41

    Other Essentials: -------------------------------------- 42

Chapter 8: -- 43

Sample Meal Plans — 43

Chapter 9: — 49

Breakfast Recipes — 49

- Smoothies and Juices — 49
  - Banana Berry Smoothie — 49
  - Green Detox Juice — 51
- Light Breakfast Options — 53
  - Oatmeal with Fruit and Nuts — 53
  - Scrambled Eggs with Spinach — 55
- Hearty Breakfast Options — 57
  - Breakfast Burrito — 57
  - Veggie Omelette — 59

Chapter 10: — 63

Lunch Recipes — 63

- Soups and Salads — 63
  - Chicken and Rice Soup — 63
  - Quinoa Salad with Vegetables — 65
- Sandwiches and Wraps — 68
  - Turkey and Avocado Wrap — 68
  - Grilled Chicken Sandwich — 69

Light Lunch Options – 72

- Cottage Cheese with Pineapple: A Refreshing Snack — 72
- Hummus and Veggie Plate: A Nutritious Powerhouse — 73

Chapter 11: — 77

Dinner Recipes – 77

Protein-Packed Dinners – 77

- Baked Salmon with Asparagus: A Light and Flavorful Meal — 77
- Grilled Chicken with Quinoa: A Protein-Packed Powerhouse — 79

Vegetarian Dinners – 82

- Stuffed Bell Peppers: A Hearty and Colorful Vegetarian Option — 82
- Lentil Stew: A Hearty and Comforting Meal 85

Chapter 12: — 88

Snack and Appetizer Recipes – 88

Quick Snacks – 88

- Shepherd's Pie vs. Turkey Meatloaf: Deciding Between Comfort Food Classics --------------------- 88

- Healthy Appetizers ------------------------------------- 91
  - Cucumber Bites with Tuna Salad: ------------ 91
  - Mini Caprese Skewers: ------------------------- 92

Indulgent Treats -- 94
  - Dark Chocolate Bark and Baked Sweet Potato Chips: A Sweet and Salty Treat --------------------- 94
  - Baked Sweet Potato Chips: ---------------------- 96

Chapter 13: -- 99

Dessert Recipes – --------------------------------------- 99

Light Desserts – -- 99
  - Yogurt Parfait with Berries: ---------------------- 99
  - Yogurt Parfait with Berries: ------------------- 100

Baked Goods – -- 103
  - Banana Bread: ----------------------------------- 103
  - Oatmeal Cookies: ------------------------------- 103

Indulgent Desserts – --------------------------------- 105
  - Chocolate Avocado Mousse: Rich and Decadent (Vegan!) ----------------------------------- 105

- Rice Pudding: Creamy Comfort Food ----- 107

INTRODUCTION

Elena looked at the blank notebook in front of her in her kitchen. The room that was once lively and happy now seemed like it was from another planet, full of uncertainty and confusion. She had a colostomy six months ago, and even though she was physically better, the emotional and dietary challenges were still hard for her.

She remembered the day she received Dr. D. Johnston's cookbook in the mail. "Nourish: A Colostomy Diet Cookbook for All" was the title, and it promised more than just recipes. It also said that it would help her get her life back. Dr. Johnston, a renowned gastroenterologist and nutritionist, had crafted the book with empathy and expertise, drawing from years of experience helping patients like Elena navigate their new normal.

When Elena opened the book, she saw a friendly note from Dr. Johnston. It wasn't the usual clinical start she was expecting. Instead, it was like talking to an old friend who knew how hard things were for her. Dr. Johnston shared stories of other patients, each facing their own unique journey but joined by a common thread of grit and hope.

Elena's eyes welled up as she read about Sarah, a young mother who found ways to prepare nutritious meals while juggling the demands of parenting and recovery. She read about Michael, a retired chef who found his love of cooking again through the book's recipes. Each story was an ode to the changing power of food and the human spirit.

These stories made Elena want to start with a simple recipe, like the Banana Berry Smoothie. The ingredients were comfortable and familiar. She followed the step-by-step instructions, appreciating the tips Dr. Johnston had included to manage gas and avoid discomfort. As she blended the bananas and berries, the vibrant colors brought a smile to her face—a small but significant victory.

The first sip of the drink was more than just a taste; it was a memory of what she could still enjoy. It was the beginning of her healing journey. Encouraged, she tried other recipes: the Quinoa Salad with Vegetables for lunch and the Baked Salmon with Asparagus for dinner. Each meal was a discovery, teaching her how to feed her body without fear.

But the guide offered more than ideas. It offered useful tips on food planning, amount control, and handling eating problems specific to colostomy patients. Dr. Johnston's caring advice helped Elena understand her body's new needs. She learned which foods to avoid and which ones to accept, slowly rebuilding her trust in the kitchen.

The parts on life with a colostomy and mental well-being were particularly helpful. Dr. Johnston emphasized the value of community and support, pushing people to connect with others who shared their experiences. Elena joined an online support group mentioned in the book, finding comfort in the shared stories and help from fellow members.

As weeks turned into months, Elena noticed major changes. She felt more active, her stomach problems were under control, and she no longer feared mealtimes. The recipe had become her beloved friend, leading her through each step of her healing.

One day, while making a batch of Oatmeal Cookies, Elena understood just how far she had come. She was no longer just living; she was thriving. The kitchen, once a place of fear and confusion, had become a haven of mending and creation.

Elena knew she had Dr. Johnston and his recipes to thank for this change. The careful meals and caring tips had enabled her to take control of her health and regain the joy of eating. She was healed, not just in body, but in spirit.

In the final part of the book, Dr. Johnston's message struck strongly with her: "This journey is not just about food; it's about finding hope and strength within yourself. You are not alone, and with each meal, you are feeding your body and soul."

Elena closed the book, her heart filled with thanks. She was ready to embrace life anew, one delicious, nourishing meal at a time.

Chapter 1:

Welcome Message

The Purpose of This Cookbook

Without the exact guide in hand, it's hard to say for certain what its goal is. However, recipes can have a variety of goals, here are a few possibilities:

- To present a specific cuisine: The book might focus on regional foods from a particular country or culture, trying to teach readers about its unique tastes and ingredients.

- To cater to a specific nutritional need: The recipes might be created for vegetarians, vegans, people with gluten intolerance, or those following a particular living diet (e.g., keto, paleo).

- To focus on a particular food skill or technique: The book could aim to teach readers about advanced culinary methods like bread making, charcuterie, or molecular gastronomy.

- To be a gathering of family favorites: The recipes might be passed down through generations, giving a comfortable and familiar approach to cooking.
- To feature seasonal ingredients: The book could showcase meals that utilize fresh, local fruit available at different times of the year.
- To be a beginner's guide to cooking: The recipes might be simple and clear, giving a basis for building kitchen confidence.

How to Use This Cookbook

Similar to the goal, the way you use a guide relies on its style and method. Here are some general tips:

- Read the opening: As mentioned before, the opening often lays out the cookbook's purpose, target audience, and any special directions or cooking tips the author wants to convey.
- Browse the Recipes: Look for foods that pique your interest or fit your wants. Consider things like food type (appetizer, main course, treat), dietary restrictions, cooking time, and item availability.

- Pay Attention to Difficulty Levels: Some guides show recipe difficulty levels (starter, middle, advanced) to help you choose suitable tasks.
- Read the Recipe Thoroughly Before Starting: Understanding the entire process beforehand helps ensure you have all the necessary items and tools, and allows you to plan your cooking flow.
- Utilize the Substitutions Section (if provided): This area can offer different items if you're missing something or have food restrictions.
- Don't Be Afraid to Experiment: While following recipes is a good starting point, feel free to change tastes, serving sizes, and presentations to fit your preferences.
- Take Notes: As you cook, jot down any changes you make or notes about the recipe's result. This personalizes the guide and helps you improve meals for future reference.

Chapter 2:

Understanding a Colostomy

A colostomy is a medical operation that makes a hole (stoma) in the belly to remove waste (stool) from the colon. The surgeon pulls a healthy piece of the colon through the abdominal wall and makes the hole. Waste then leaves the body through the stoma into a storage pouch worn on the belly.

Types of Colostomies

There are two main types of colostomies:

- **Temporary Colostomy:** This type is used to allow the sick or damaged part of the colon to heal. After healing, another surgery can reverse the colostomy, rejoining the colon and allowing waste to pass through the rectum again.
- **Permanent Colostomy:** This type is necessary when the colon cannot work properly, or if it has been removed due to disease or accident.

There are also different types of colostomies based on the position of the stoma on the colon:

- **Ileostomy:** This produces a hole from the end of the small intestine (ileum) instead of the colon. It's a different process but serves a similar purpose.

Common Concerns After Colostomy Surgery

- **Stoma Care:** Learning proper cleaning and care of the stoma and collection pouch is crucial to avoid infection and leaking.
- **Body Image:** Some people experience mental issues changing to their body after surgery.
- **Diet and Lifestyle:** Dietary changes may be necessary to control waste uniformity and avoid clogs. Most people can return to most tasks after healing.

Myths About Colostomies

Myth: People with colostomies cannot live a normal life.

Reality: With proper care and control, most people with colostomies can lead full and busy lives.

Myth: Colostomies are embarrassing and noticeable.

Reality: Pouches are meant to be covert and odor-proof.

Myth: People with colostomies cannot move or swim.

Reality: With proper planning and stoma care, these things are possible.

Chapter 3:
Nutrition Basics

Importance of a Balanced Diet for Colostomy Patients

A healthy diet is important for everyone, but it holds special importance for people who have undergone a colostomy. Here's why:

- Healing and Recovery: After surgery, your body needs proper diet to heal the wound and support general well-being. A healthy diet offers the necessary building blocks for muscle repair and defense function.
- Nutrient Absorption: Depending on the position of the colostomy, some gut processes might be skipped. A varied diet ensures you're getting a variety of nutrients your body might not be receiving as efficiently.
- Stoma Function: Certain foods can affect the regularity and flow of your stoma. A healthy diet helps control gas, bloating, constipation, and diarrhea, supporting reliable and easy gut function.

- Energy Levels: Maintaining a healthy diet ensures you have the energy to go about your daily tasks and improves general well-being.

Key Nutrients for Colostomy Patients

Here are some key nutrients to consider in your diet after a colostomy:

- Protein: Crucial for making and mending cells. Aim for lean protein sources like fish, chicken, beans, and lentils.
- Fluids: Dehydration can increase constipation. Drink plenty of water throughout the day, especially after colostomy surgery.
- Electrolytes: Electrolytes like sodium and potassium are lost in stool output. Consider adding broths, sports drinks, and foods like bananas to refill them.
- Fiber: Fiber helps control bowel movements and supports gut health. Aim for a reasonable amount from sources like whole grains, fruits, and veggies. However, some high-fiber choices might need to be introduced gradually or avoided originally to handle gas and bloating.

Consult your doctor or a certified nutritionist for specific suggestions.
- Healthy Fats: Include healthy fats from sources like eggs, nuts, and olive oil in your diet. These increase nutrient intake and satisfaction.

Chapter 4:

Colostomy Diet Principles

Foods to Avoid After Colostomy Surgery

Here's a list of things that might be best to avoid or reduce immediately after colostomy surgery, or if they cause gas or stomach issues:

High-Fiber Foods: While fiber is usually important, some high-fiber choices can cause gas and bloating, especially in the initial healing phase. This includes:

Raw veggies like broccoli, cauliflower, cabbage, Brussels sprouts, and onions

Whole foods like brown rice, whole-wheat bread, and quinoa

Dried fruits like raisins and prunes

Legumes like beans, lentils, and peas

Spicy Foods: Spicy foods can upset the digestive system and increase gas or diarrhea.

Fatty Foods: Fried foods and fatty meats can be difficult to digest and might add to constipation.

- **Carbonated Drinks:** The carbonation can cause gas and bloating.
- **Dairy Products (if Lactose Intolerant):** Lactose intolerance can lead to bloating, gas, and diarrhea. If you suspect lactose intolerance, try lactose-free dairy goods or replacements.
- **Alcohol:** Alcohol can dehydrate you and possibly upset the digestive system.
- **Caffeine:** Excessive caffeine might lead to diarrhea.
- **Sugar Alcohols**: Found in sugar-free sweets and chewing gum, sugar alcohols can cause gas and bloating.

Foods to Include After Colostomy Surgery

Focus on easily edible and nutritious foods that support good gut function and general well-being. Here are some good options:

- Lean Protein Sources: Fish, chicken, eggs, and lean cuts of meat provide necessary protein for healing and keeping muscle strength.

- Well-Cooked Vegetables: Steamed or cooked veggies are easier to digest and provide important vitamins and minerals.
- Ripe Fruits: Bananas, mangoes, and applesauce are good sources of vitamins, minerals, and water.
- Refined Grains: White rice, white bread, and pasta are easier to digest than whole grains initially.
- Probiotics: Yogurt with live and active bacteria can improve gut health and possibly reduce bloating.

Managing Gas and Odor

Gas and stink are usual issues after colostomy surgery. Here are some tips for handling them:

- **Eat Smaller Meals More Frequently:** This can help your digestive system handle food more effectively and reduce gas buildup.
- **Chew Thoroughly:** This allows for better food breakdown and lowers the amount of air swallowed while eating.
- **Identify and Limit Gas-Producing Foods:** Pay attention to how your body responds to certain things and change your diet accordingly.
- **Stay Hydrated**: Drinking plenty of water helps move stool through your system and can reduce gas.
- **Consider Activated Charcoal:** Talk to your doctor about whether activated charcoal tablets might be appropriate to help absorb gas in your digestive system.
- **Use Odor-Controlling Products**: Odor-proof mouth covers and deodorizing sprays can help control odor issues.

Hydration Tips

Staying wet is important for general health and proper stoma function. Here are some tips:

- **Drink plenty of water throughout the day: Aim** for 8-10 glasses of water everyday, or more if you're busy or sweating.
- **Choose hydrating beverages**: Water, herbal drinks, broths, and reduced fruit juices are good choices.
- **Eat water-rich fruits and vegetables:** Watermelon, cucumber, and celery can add to your fluid diet.
- **Monitor your pee color**: Pale yellow pee shows good hydration, while dark yellow urine suggests dehydration.

Chapter 5:
Special Considerations

Managing Diarrhea After Colostomy Surgery

Diarrhea is a usual worry after colostomy surgery, especially during the initial healing phase. Here are some tips for handling it:

- Stay Hydrated: Dehydration can worsen diarrhea. Drink plenty of fluids like water, clear broths, and vitamin drinks to replace fluids lost in stool output.
- BRAT Diet: This boring diet (Bananas, Rice, Applesauce, and Toast) is easily edible and can help firm up stools.
- Probiotics: Consider including yogurt with live and active cultures or probiotic pills to support gut health and possibly reduce diarrhea.
- Medication: Antidiarrheal medicines might be given by your doctor to control serious or chronic diarrhea.

Managing Constipation After Colostomy Surgery

Constipation can also occur after colostomy surgery. Here are some tips for handling it:

- Increase Fiber Intake (gradually): Fiber helps add bulk to stool and promotes bowel movements. However, add high-fiber foods gradually to avoid excessive gas and bloating. Start with well-cooked or canned veggies, and gradually add fruits and whole grains.
- Hydration: Drinking plenty of water throughout the day softens stool and makes it easier to pass.
- Exercise: Regular physical exercise boosts your gut system and can help avoid constipation.
- Laxatives: If food changes and water aren't sufficient, your doctor might suggest a stool softener or laxative.

Dealing with Blockages (Stoma Obstruction)

A stoma blockage (bowel obstruction) is a dangerous problem that needs quick medical care. Here are some signs to watch for:

Abdominal pain and cramping

Swelling or pain in the belly

Nausea and vomiting

Reduced or no flow from the stoma

Inability to pass gas

If you experience any of these signs, do not try to treat the blockage yourself. Seek quick medical care from your doctor or emergency room.

Here are some protective steps to lower the chance of blockages:

- Chew food thoroughly: This allows for better digestion and lowers the risk of big food pieces getting stuck in your stoma.
- Stay hydrated: Drinking plenty of water helps keep stool soft and easy to pass through the stoma.

- Eat a healthy diet: Include fiber-rich foods gradually, as directed by your doctor, to promote normal bowel movements.
- Avoid certain foods: Limit or avoid foods that frequently cause constipation or clogs, such as corn, nuts, and dried fruits

Chapter 6:

Post-Surgery Diet Phases

Initial Post-Surgery Diet (First Few Weeks)

The initial post-colostomy diet focuses on promoting healing and reducing stomach pain. Here's what you might expect:

Clear Liquids: Immediately after surgery, you might start with clear liquids like water, soup, clear fruit drinks (apple, grape), to ensure you can handle fluids without sickness or puking.

Bland, Low-Fiber Foods: Once you accept clear drinks, your doctor will likely introduce a bland, low-fiber diet. This might include:

White bread, toast, or crackers

White rice or pasta

Well-cooked or canned veggies (peeled potatoes, carrots)

Lean protein sources (skinless chicken breast, baked fish)

Ripe veggies (applesauce, bananas)

Smooth nut butters (skip thick types)

Small Frequent Meals: Eating smaller meals more frequently (6 small meals instead of 3 big ones) can help ease digestion and reduce bloating.

Transitioning to a Regular Diet (After a Few Weeks)

As you heal and your gut system changes, you can gradually move to a more normal diet. Here are some tips:

Reintroduce Foods Slowly: Start with one new food at a time and watch your body's response. Wait a few days before offering another new food.

Focus on Balance: Aim for a healthy meal that includes:

Lean protein sources

Whole grains (gradually increase quantity)

A range of fruits and veggies (cooked or raw based on ability)

Healthy fats (avocado, olive oil)

Maintain Hydration: Continue to drink plenty of water throughout the day.

Listen to Your Body: Pay attention to how you feel after eating certain things. If you experience gas, bloating, diarrhea, or constipation, it might be best to limit or avoid that specific food.

Long-Term Dietary Adjustments

While you can usually return to most foods after colostomy surgery, some long-term dietary changes might be beneficial:

- Fiber Intake: Fiber is important for gut health, but it can also cause gas and bloating. Aim for a modest amount of fiber and choose low-FODMAP choices (ask a nutritionist for a list) initially. Gradually increase fiber intake as allowed.
- Gas-Producing Foods: Certain foods like beans, cabbage, and broccoli might cause extra gas. Limit these or discover your individual triggers and change accordingly.
- Spicy Foods: Spicy foods can upset the digestive system. Limit them if they cause pain.

- Alcohol and Caffeine: Consume these in moderation, as they might add to dehydration or diarrhea.
- Probiotics: Consider including yogurt with live and active cultures or probiotic pills to support gut health.

Chapter 7:
Meal Planning Tips

Creating a Balanced Meal Plan After Colostomy Surgery

Following a healthy meal plan is important for good health after colostomy surgery. Here's how to make one:

- Consider Your Needs: Think about your exercise level, calorie needs, and any nutritional limits. Consult a doctor or trained chef for personalized advice.
- Include All Food Groups: Aim for a balanced plate with protein, starches, fruits, veggies, and healthy fats at each meal.
- Variety is Key: Include a number of colors and tastes within each food group to ensure you're getting a wide range of minerals.
- Plan Meals and Snacks: Planning ahead helps ensure you have healthy options easily available and lowers the desire for bad choices.

- Portion Control is Key: Use smaller plates and bowls to control serving sizes. Here are some broad guidelines:
- Protein: 3-4 ounces (palm-sized amount)
- Grains: ½ cup cooked (fist-sized amount)
- Vegetables: 1 cup cooked or raw (two handfuls)
- Fruits: 1 big piece (baseball-sized)
- Healthy Fats: 1 tablespoon (thumb-sized amount)
- Sample Balanced Meal Plan: Breakfast:
- Greek yogurt with berries and a sprinkle of granola
- Scrambled eggs with whole-wheat toast and avocado slices
- **Lunch:**
- Grilled chicken breast salad with mixed greens, rice, carrots, and a light vinegar dressing
- Lentil soup with a whole-wheat roll

• Dinner:

- Baked fish with roasted veggies (broccoli, asparagus) and brown rice Turkey soup with a side salad

- **Snacks:**
  - Apple pieces with almond butter
  - Cottage cheese with sliced veggies
  - Handful of mixed nuts

Shopping List Essentials:

Here's a starting point for your shopping list, focused on post-colostomy safe options:

Protein Sources:

Lean meats (chicken breast, fish, turkey)

Eggs

Tofu or tempeh (vegetarian choice)

Low-fat yogurt or cottage cheese

Carbohydrates:

White bread, rice, and pasta (gradually add whole grains)

Oatmeal Quinoa

Sweet potatoes

Fruits:

Bananas Apples

Cantaloupe

Canned fruits (in natural juice) Vegetables:

Well-cooked or canned carrots, green beans, peas Ripe tomatoes Lettuce Spinach Healthy Fats:

Olive oil Avocado Nuts and nut butters (smooth types)

Other Essentials:

Low-fiber crackers

Broth Clear broths and drinks (for initial healing)

Probiotic yogurt (if allowed)

Plenty of water

Chapter 8:
Sample Meal Plans

Day 1:

- **Breakfast:** Scrambled eggs with chopped spinach and a slice of whole-wheat toast
- **Lunch:** Chicken breast salad with mixed greens, diced avocado, and a light vinaigrette dressing. Whole-wheat crackers on the side.
- **Dinner:** Baked salmon with roasted asparagus and brown rice.
- **Snacks (choose 2):** Apple slices with almond butter, banana with a sprinkle of cinnamon, Greek yogurt with berries.

Day 2:

- **Breakfast:** Oatmeal with sliced banana and a drizzle of honey.
- **Lunch:** Lentil soup with a side salad (mixed greens, cherry tomatoes, light vinaigrette).

- **Dinner:** Turkey chili with a dollop of low-fat Greek yogurt and a side of steamed broccoli.

- **Snacks (choose 2):** Cottage cheese with sliced cucumber, pear with string cheese, handful of mixed nuts.

Day 3:

- **Breakfast:** Smoothie made with Greek yogurt, banana, spinach, and a splash of milk.

- **Lunch:** Tuna salad sandwich on whole-wheat bread with lettuce and tomato. Carrot sticks on the side.

- **Dinner:** Baked chicken breast with mashed sweet potatoes and steamed green beans.

- **Snacks (choose 2):** Crackers with low-fat cheese, grapes with a sprinkle of sunflower seeds, rice cakes with mashed avocado.

Day 4:

- **Breakfast:** Whole-wheat pancakes with sliced banana and a drizzle of maple syrup.

- **Lunch:** Leftover chicken breast from Day 3 with a side salad and quinoa.

- **Dinner:** Poached white fish with steamed carrots and brown rice.

- **Snacks (choose 2):** Cottage cheese with sliced pineapple, whole-wheat crackers with hummus, apple slices with nut butter.

Day 5:

- **Breakfast:** Scrambled eggs with chopped tomatoes and a slice of whole-wheat toast.

- **Lunch:** Vegetarian chili with a side salad and a whole-wheat roll.

- **Dinner:** Baked salmon with roasted Brussels sprouts and quinoa.

- **Snacks (choose 2):** Pear with string cheese, handful of dried cranberries (introduce gradually), Greek yogurt with berries.

Day 6:

- **Breakfast:** Oatmeal with sliced apple and a sprinkle of chopped walnuts.

- **Lunch:** Chicken Caesar salad with grilled chicken breast, romaine lettuce, light Caesar dressing, and whole-wheat croutons (limit croutons if needed).

- **Dinner:** Turkey burgers on whole-wheat buns with sweet potato fries (baked or air-fried).

- **Snacks (choose 2):** Cottage cheese with sliced peaches, banana with a drizzle of honey, rice cakes with mashed avocado and salsa.

Day 7:

- **Breakfast:** Whole-wheat waffles with sliced banana and a dollop of low-fat yogurt.

- **Lunch:** Leftover turkey burger from Day 6 with a side salad.

- **Dinner:** Baked chicken breast with roasted vegetables (broccoli, zucchini) and brown rice.

- **Snacks (choose 2):** Apple slices with almond butter, pear with string cheese, handful of mixed nuts.

7-Day Meal Plan for Advanced Diets:

Day 1 (Gluten-Free):

- **Breakfast:** Chia seed pudding with almond milk, berries, and chopped nuts.

- **Lunch:** Grilled salmon with quinoa salad (quinoa, chopped vegetables, herbs, olive oil dressing).

- **Dinner:** Coconut curry chicken with brown rice noodles and roasted green beans.

- **Snacks (choose 2):** Apple slices with almond butter, vegetable sticks with hummus, protein shake with almond milk and berries.

Day 2 (Vegetarian):

- **Breakfast:** Tofu scramble with chopped vegetables and whole-wheat toast.

- **Lunch:** Lentil soup with a side salad (mixed greens, avocado, balsamic vinaigrette).

- **Dinner:** Vegetarian chili with brown rice and a dollop of Greek yogurt.

- **Snacks (choose 2):** Edamame pods, cottage cheese with sliced cucumber and tomatoes, fruit salad with a drizzle of honey.

Day 3 (High-Protein):

- **Breakfast:** Greek yogurt with berries, granola, and a scoop of protein powder.

Chapter 9:

Breakfast Recipes

Smoothies and Juices

• Banana Berry Smoothie

This refreshing and nutritious smoothie is a great way to incorporate fruits and yogurt into your diet.

Ingredients (Serves 1):

- 1 medium banana, frozen
- 1 cup mixed berries (fresh or frozen)
- 1/2 cup plain yogurt (Greek or regular)
- 1/4 cup milk (dairy or plant-based)
- Optional: Honey or maple syrup to taste (for additional sweetness)

Instructions:

1. Blend all ingredients together in a blender until smooth and creamy.

2. Add more milk or water for a thinner consistency, or add more frozen banana for a thicker consistency.

3. Enjoy immediately!

Nutritional Information (approximate values per serving):

- Calories: 250-300 (depending on yogurt and milk type)
- Carbohydrates: 40-50 grams
- Protein: 10-15 grams
- Fat: 3-5 grams
- Fiber: 4-6 grams
- Vitamins and minerals: Vitamin C, potassium, calcium (depending on ingredients)

Tips:

- You can use any type of berries you like, such as strawberries, blueberries, raspberries, or blackberries.
- If you don't have fresh berries, frozen berries work well too.

- For a thicker smoothie, use all frozen fruit.

- Add a scoop of protein powder for an extra protein boost.

- For a vegan option, use plant-based yogurt and milk.

• Green Detox Juice

Ingredients (Serves 1):

- 1 cucumber, peeled and chopped

- 1 celery stalk, chopped

- 1 apple, cored and chopped (optional)

- 1/2 lemon, juiced

- 1 handful spinach or kale

- Optional: Ginger knob, peeled and chopped (for a spicy kick)

Instructions:

1. Wash all produce thoroughly.

2. Juice all ingredients using a juicer.

3. If the juice is too strong, dilute it with a little water.

4. Enjoy immediately!

Nutritional Information (approximate values per serving):

- Calories: 50-70
- Carbohydrates: 10-15 grams
- Protein: 1-2 grams
- Fat: less than 1 gram
- Fiber: 2-3 grams
- Vitamins and minerals: Vitamin A, Vitamin C, potassium, iron (depending on ingredients)

Tips:

- You can adjust the ingredients to your taste. For example, if you don't like cucumber, you can use more apple or another fruit.
- If you don't have a juicer, you can blend the ingredients together and then strain out the pulp.

- It's best to drink green juice fresh for the most nutrients.

Time per Serving:

- Smoothie: 2-3 minutes (blending time)
- Green Juice: 5-7 minutes (prep and juicing time)

Light Breakfast Options

• Oatmeal with Fruit and Nuts

Oatmeal is a classic and healthy breakfast option that's easily customizable. Here's a basic recipe with some variations:

Ingredients (Serves 1):

- 1/2 cup rolled oats (or quick oats for faster cooking)
- 1 cup water or milk (dairy or plant-based)
- Pinch of salt (optional)
- Toppings (choose your favorites):

- Fresh or frozen fruit (berries, banana, mango)
- Nuts and seeds (sliced almonds, chopped walnuts, chia seeds)
- Spices (cinnamon, nutmeg)
- Sweetener (honey, maple syrup, brown sugar)

Instructions:

1. In a saucepan, combine oats, water/milk, and salt (if using).
2. Bring to a boil over medium heat, then reduce heat and simmer for 5-7 minutes (or according to package instructions) for rolled oats, or 1-2 minutes for quick oats, stirring occasionally.
3. Remove from heat and let sit for a minute or two to thicken further.
4. Add your chosen toppings and enjoy!

Variations:

- **Creamy Oatmeal:** Add a splash of cream cheese, yogurt, or nut butter to the cooked oatmeal for extra richness.

- **Baked Oatmeal:** Combine rolled oats, milk, fruit, nuts, and spices in a baking dish. Bake in a preheated oven at 375°F (190°C) for 20-25 minutes, or until set.

- **Overnight Oats:** Combine rolled oats, milk, yogurt, and chia seeds in a jar. Refrigerate overnight for a grab-and-go breakfast.

• Scrambled Eggs with Spinach

Scrambled eggs are another quick and versatile breakfast option. Adding spinach provides a boost of nutrients.

Ingredients (Serves 1):

- 2 eggs
- 1 tablespoon milk (dairy or plant-based)
- 1/2 cup fresh spinach, chopped
- 1 tablespoon butter or olive oil
- Salt and pepper to taste

- Optional additions:
    - Chopped vegetables (onion, bell peppers, mushrooms)
    - Cheese (shredded cheddar, feta, goat cheese)
    - Chopped herbs (fresh parsley, chives)

Instructions:

1. In a bowl, whisk together eggs and milk.
2. Heat butter or oil in a pan over medium heat.
3. Add chopped vegetables (if using) and cook until softened.
4. Add spinach and cook until wilted.
5. Pour in the egg mixture and scramble with a spatula until cooked through to your desired consistency.
6. Season with salt and pepper to taste.
7. Remove from heat and serve immediately.
8. Top with cheese, herbs, or other desired ingredients (optional).

Tips:

- For fluffier scrambled eggs, separate the eggs and whisk the whites until stiff peaks form. Then, gently fold the whites into the yolk mixture.

- Don't overcook the eggs, as they will become tough.

Hearty Breakfast Options

• Breakfast Burrito

A breakfast burrito is a complete and portable breakfast option. Here's a basic recipe with vegetarian and protein-packed variations:

Ingredients (Serves 1):

- 1 large flour tortilla
- 2 scrambled eggs (see recipe above)
- 1/2 cup shredded cheese (cheddar, Monterey Jack, or your favorite)
- Other fillings (choose your favorites):

- Cooked black beans or pinto beans
- Sliced avocado
- Chopped salsa
- Diced tomatoes
- Sauteed vegetables (onions, peppers, mushrooms)
- Cooked breakfast sausage or chorizo (for non-vegetarian option)

Instructions:

1. Warm the tortilla in a dry skillet or microwave for a few seconds to make it pliable.
2. Scramble your eggs according to the recipe above.
3. Spread a layer of scrambled eggs onto the warmed tortilla.
4. Add your chosen fillings in layers.
5. Fold the bottom edge of the tortilla over the filling, then fold in the sides. Roll up tightly.
6. Serve immediately and enjoy!

Variations:

- **Vegetarian Protein Powerhouse:** Add scrambled tofu or tempeh instead of eggs, along with black beans, salsa, avocado, and sauteed vegetables.

- **Spicy Chorizo Scramble:** Saute diced chorizo in a pan, then scramble eggs with the chorizo. Add cheese, salsa, and other desired fillings.

• Veggie Omelette

Ingredients (Serves 1):

- 2 eggs
- 1 tablespoon milk (dairy or plant-based)
- Pinch of salt and pepper
- 1/4 cup chopped vegetables (spinach, mushrooms, onions, peppers)
- 1/4 cup shredded cheese (optional)
- 1 tablespoon butter or olive oil

Instructions:

1. In a bowl, whisk together eggs, milk, salt, and pepper.//
2. Heat butter or oil in a pan over medium heat.
3. Add chopped vegetables and cook until softened.
4. Pour in the egg mixture, swirling the pan to coat the bottom evenly.
5. As the omelette cooks, gently lift the edges with a spatula to allow the uncooked egg to flow underneath.
6. Sprinkle cheese over one half of the omelette (if using).
7. Once cooked through (set on the bottom and slightly loose on top), fold the other half of the omelette over the cheese using a spatula.
8. Serve immediately and enjoy!

Variations:

- **Hearty Veggie Scramble:** If you prefer scrambled eggs instead of an omelette, simply pour the egg mixture over the cooked vegetables and scramble until set.

- **Mediterranean Delight:** Add chopped sun-dried tomatoes, crumbled feta cheese, and chopped olives to your omelette.

- **Spicy Fiesta:** Saute diced jalapenos along with other vegetables for a kick. Top with salsa and avocado.

Chapter 10:

Lunch Recipes –

Soups and Salads –

• Chicken and Rice Soup

This comforting chicken and rice soup is a classic for a reason! It's easy to make, packed with flavor, and perfect for a light meal or a satisfying starter.

Ingredients (Serves 4-6):

- 1 tablespoon olive oil
- 1 medium onion, chopped
- 2 carrots, chopped
- 2 celery stalks, chopped
- 4 cloves garlic, minced
- 8 cups chicken broth
- 1 pound boneless, skinless chicken breasts or thighs, cut into bite-sized pieces

- 1 cup uncooked white rice
- 1/2 teaspoon dried thyme
- 1/4 teaspoon salt
- 1/4 teaspoon black pepper
- Optional additions:
    - 1 cup frozen peas
    - 1/2 cup chopped fresh parsley
    - Cooked shredded chicken (leftovers work great!)

Instructions:

1. Heat olive oil in a large pot over medium heat.
2. Add onion, carrots, and celery. Cook for 5-7 minutes, or until softened.
3. Add garlic and cook for an additional minute, stirring frequently.
4. Pour in chicken broth and bring to a boil.
5. Add chicken pieces, thyme, salt, and pepper. Reduce heat to simmer and cook for 15-20 minutes, or until chicken is cooked through.

6. Stir in rice and simmer for another 15-20 minutes, or until rice is cooked and fluffy.

7. Add frozen peas (if using) and cook for an additional 2-3 minutes, or until heated through.

8. Remove from heat and stir in chopped parsley (if using).

9. Serve hot and enjoy!

Tips:

- For a richer flavor, you can brown the chicken pieces in the pot before adding the vegetables.

- You can use brown rice instead of white rice for added fiber. However, adjust the cooking time according to package instructions.

- Leftovers can be stored in an airtight container in the refrigerator for up to 3 days.

• Quinoa Salad with Vegetables

This quinoa salad is a light and refreshing side dish that's packed with nutrients and flavor. It's perfect for a healthy lunch or a potluck contribution.

Ingredients (Serves 4-6):

- 1 cup quinoa, rinsed
- 1 1/2 cups water or chicken broth
- 1 cucumber, diced
- 1 red bell pepper, diced
- 1/2 cup cherry tomatoes, halved
- 1/4 cup crumbled feta cheese (optional)
- 1/4 cup chopped fresh parsley
- 2 tablespoons olive oil
- 1 tablespoon lemon juice
- Salt and pepper to taste

Instructions:

1. In a saucepan, combine quinoa and water/broth. Bring to a boil, then reduce heat to low, cover, and simmer for 15-20 minutes, or until quinoa is cooked and fluffy. Fluff with a fork and let cool slightly.

2. In a large bowl, combine cooked quinoa, diced cucumber, red bell pepper, cherry tomatoes, and feta cheese (if using).

3. In a small bowl, whisk together olive oil, lemon juice, salt, and pepper.

4. Pour the dressing over the quinoa and vegetable mixture and toss to coat evenly.

5. Garnish with chopped fresh parsley and serve.

Tips:

- You can add other vegetables to this salad, such as chopped corn, chopped zucchini, or black beans.

- If you don't have fresh parsley, you can use another herb, such as dill or cilantro.

- Leftovers can be stored in an airtight container in the refrigerator for up to 3 days.

Sandwiches and Wraps –

• Turkey and Avocado Wrap

This wrap is a healthy and satisfying lunch option that's packed with protein and flavor.

Ingredients (Serves 1):

- 1 large whole wheat tortilla
- 4-5 slices thinly sliced turkey breast
- 1/4 avocado, sliced
- 1/2 cup mixed greens
- 1 tomato, sliced
- 1 tablespoon light mayonnaise (or hummus for a vegan option)
- Salt and pepper to taste
- Optional additions:
    - Shredded cheese
    - Sliced red onion
    - Chopped cucumber

- Dijon mustard

Instructions:

1. Spread mayonnaise (or hummus) evenly on the whole wheat tortilla.

2. Layer turkey slices, avocado slices, mixed greens, and tomato slices on the tortilla.

3. Season with salt and pepper to taste.

4. Add any optional ingredients you like.

5. Fold the bottom edge of the tortilla up over the filling. Then, fold in the sides tightly. Roll up the tortilla securely.

6. Cut the wrap in half and enjoy!

• Grilled Chicken Sandwich

This classic sandwich is a delicious and versatile option for lunch or dinner.

Ingredients (Serves 1):

- 1 boneless, skinless chicken breast
- 1 tablespoon olive oil

- 1/2 teaspoon dried thyme
- 1/4 teaspoon salt
- 1/4 teaspoon black pepper
- 2 slices whole wheat bread
- Lettuce, tomato, and onion (optional)
- Mayonnaise, mustard, or your favorite sauce (optional)

Instructions:

1. Marinate the chicken breast: In a bowl, combine olive oil, thyme, salt, and pepper. Add the chicken breast and coat it evenly with the marinade. Marinate for at least 15 minutes or up to 30 minutes for extra flavor.
2. Preheat a grill pan or grill to medium heat.
3. Grill the chicken breast for 5-7 minutes per side, or until cooked through.
4. While the chicken is cooking, toast the bread slices if desired.
5. Spread your favorite sauce on the toasted bread slices (optional).

6. Place the cooked chicken breast on one slice of bread.

7. Add lettuce, tomato, and onion slices (optional) to the sandwich.

8. Top with the other slice of bread and enjoy!

Tips:

- You can grill the chicken breast on a stovetop grill pan or on an outdoor grill.

- You can adjust the cooking time for the chicken breast depending on its thickness.

- Get creative with your sandwich fillings! You can add cheese, avocado, pickles, or other condiments to your liking.

- For a healthier option, skip the mayo or use a light mayo option.

Light Lunch Options –

• Cottage Cheese with Pineapple: A Refreshing Snack

Cottage cheese with pineapple is a light and refreshing snack that's perfect for a hot day or whenever you need a protein boost. It's also a good option for a post-surgery meal as it's easy to digest.

Ingredients (Serves 1):

- 1/2 cup low-fat cottage cheese
- 1/4 cup chopped fresh pineapple
- 1 tablespoon chopped nuts or seeds (optional)
- Drizzle of honey or maple syrup (optional)
- Fresh mint leaves for garnish (optional)

Instructions:

1. In a bowl, combine cottage cheese and chopped pineapple.
2. Top with chopped nuts or seeds for added texture and healthy fats (optional).

3. Drizzle with a touch of honey or maple syrup for additional sweetness (optional).

4. Garnish with fresh mint leaves for a refreshing touch (optional).

• Hummus and Veggie Plate: A Nutritious Powerhouse

Hummus and veggie plate is a colorful, flavorful, and nutritious snack or light meal option. It provides protein from the hummus, fiber and vitamins from the vegetables, and healthy fats from the olive oil in the hummus.

Ingredients (Serves 1):

- 1/3 cup hummus (variety of flavors available)
- Selection of raw vegetables (choose your favorites):
    - Baby carrots
    - Cherry tomatoes
    - Cucumber slices
    - Bell pepper strips

- Celery sticks
- Broccoli florets
- Sugar snap peas
* Extra virgin olive oil for drizzling (optional)
* Sprinkle of dried herbs (optional)

Instructions:

1. Arrange your chosen raw vegetables on a plate.
2. Serve the hummus in a small bowl alongside the vegetables.
3. Drizzle a few drops of olive oil over the vegetables for extra flavor (optional).
4. Sprinkle with dried herbs like oregano or parsley for an extra touch (optional).

Tips:

* For the veggie plate, choose a variety of colors and textures for a more visually appealing and interesting snack.
* Pre-cut vegetables can save you time and make this snack option even more convenient.

- If you don't have fresh herbs, a pinch of salt and pepper can also add some flavor to the vegetables.

- For a heartier option, serve whole-wheat crackers or pita bread wedges alongside the hummus and veggies.

Chapter 11:

Dinner Recipes –

Protein-Packed Dinners –

• Baked Salmon with Asparagus: A Light and Flavorful Meal

Baked salmon with asparagus is a classic and healthy dish that's perfect for a weeknight meal. It's easy to prepare, requires minimal cleanup, and provides a good dose of protein and omega-3 fatty acids.

Ingredients (Serves 2):

- 2 salmon fillets (each about 6 ounces)
- 1 tablespoon olive oil
- 1/2 teaspoon dried thyme
- 1/4 teaspoon salt
- 1/4 teaspoon black pepper
- 1 bunch asparagus, trimmed

- Lemon wedges (optional)

Instructions:

1. Preheat oven to 400°F (200°C).

2. In a small bowl, combine olive oil, thyme, salt, and pepper.

3. Place salmon fillets in a baking dish. Brush the salmon with the olive oil mixture, coating both sides.

4. Arrange the asparagus spears alongside the salmon in the baking dish. You can drizzle the asparagus with a little olive oil as well (optional).

5. Bake for 15-20 minutes, or until the salmon is cooked through and flakes easily with a fork. The asparagus should be tender-crisp.

6. Serve immediately with lemon wedges for squeezing over the fish if desired.

• Grilled Chicken with Quinoa: A Protein-Packed Powerhouse

Grilled chicken with quinoa is a delicious and nutritious meal that's perfect for a lunch or dinner. It's packed with protein from the chicken and quinoa, and you can customize it with your favorite vegetables and seasonings.

Ingredients (Serves 2):

- 2 boneless, skinless chicken breasts
- 1 tablespoon olive oil
- 1/2 teaspoon dried oregano
- 1/4 teaspoon salt
- 1/4 teaspoon black pepper
- 1 cup quinoa, rinsed
- 1 1/2 cups chicken broth or water
- 1 cup chopped vegetables (optional - bell peppers, onions, zucchini)
- 1/4 cup chopped fresh parsley (optional)

Instructions:

For the Chicken:

1. In a bowl, combine olive oil, oregano, salt, and pepper.

2. Marinate the chicken breasts in the mixture for at least 15 minutes or up to 30 minutes for extra flavor.

3. Preheat a grill pan or outdoor grill to medium heat.

4. Grill the chicken breasts for 5-7 minutes per side, or until cooked through.

For the Quinoa:

1. While the chicken is cooking, cook the quinoa according to package instructions. In a saucepan, combine quinoa and chicken broth or water. Bring to a boil, then reduce heat to low, cover, and simmer for 15-20 minutes, or until quinoa is cooked and fluffy. Fluff with a fork.

Assemble the Meal:

1. Plate the cooked quinoa.

2. Top with the grilled chicken breast.

3. Add chopped vegetables (if using) to the quinoa for extra flavor and nutrients.

4. Garnish with fresh parsley (optional).

Tips:

- You can marinate the chicken in your favorite marinade instead of using the suggested ingredients.

- If you don't have a grill pan, you can cook the chicken breasts in a skillet over medium heat.

- For a vegetarian option, replace the chicken with tofu or tempeh, marinated and grilled in the same way.

Vegetarian Dinners –

• Stuffed Bell Peppers: A Hearty and Colorful Vegetarian Option

Stuffed bell peppers are a versatile and delicious dish that can be enjoyed hot or cold. This recipe uses lentils for a protein and fiber-rich vegetarian filling.

Ingredients (Serves 4):

- 4 large bell peppers (any color combination)
- 1 cup cooked brown lentils (or 1/2 cup dry lentils, cooked according to package instructions)
- 1 cup cooked brown rice (or 1/2 cup dry brown rice, cooked according to package instructions)
- 1 medium onion, diced
- 1 clove garlic, minced
- 1 cup chopped vegetables (such as mushrooms, carrots, celery)
- 1 can (14.5 oz) diced tomatoes, undrained

- 1/2 cup vegetable broth

- 1/4 cup chopped fresh parsley

- 1/4 cup grated Parmesan cheese (optional)

- 2 tablespoons olive oil

- Salt and pepper to taste

Instructions:

1. Preheat oven to 375°F (190°C).

2. Prepare the bell peppers: Wash the bell peppers and cut off the tops, leaving the stems on for presentation (optional). Carefully remove the seeds and membranes from the inside.

3. Cook the filling: In a large skillet, heat olive oil over medium heat. Add diced onion and cook until softened, about 5 minutes.

4. Add minced garlic and cook for an additional minute, stirring frequently.

5. Add chopped vegetables and cook until softened, about 5-7 minutes.

6. Stir in cooked lentils, cooked brown rice, diced tomatoes with their juices, and vegetable broth.

7. Bring to a simmer and cook for 5 minutes, or until the mixture thickens slightly.

8. Season with salt and pepper to taste.

9. Stir in chopped fresh parsley.

10. Stuffing the peppers: Spoon the lentil mixture evenly into the prepared bell peppers. Top with grated Parmesan cheese (optional).

11. Place the stuffed peppers in a baking dish. Add about 1/4 cup of water to the bottom of the dish to prevent sticking.

12. Bake for 30-35 minutes, or until the bell peppers are tender and the filling is heated through.

13. Serve hot, warm, or at room temperature.

• Lentil Stew: A Hearty and Comforting Meal

Lentil stew is a classic and cozy dish that's perfect for a cold day. It's packed with protein and fiber from the lentils, and you can customize it with your favorite vegetables and spices.

Ingredients (Serves 4-6):

- 1 tablespoon olive oil
- 1 medium onion, diced
- 2 carrots, diced
- 2 celery stalks, diced
- 2 cloves garlic, minced
- 1 teaspoon ground cumin
- 1/2 teaspoon dried thyme
- 1/4 teaspoon red pepper flakes (optional)
- 1 cup brown lentils, rinsed
- 4 cups vegetable broth
- 1 can (14.5 oz) diced tomatoes, undrained

- 1 cup chopped kale or spinach
- Salt and pepper to taste

Instructions:

1. In a large pot, heat olive oil over medium heat.
2. Add diced onion, carrots, and celery. Cook until softened, about 5-7 minutes.
3. Add minced garlic, cumin, thyme, and red pepper flakes (if using). Cook for an additional minute, stirring constantly, to release the fragrance of the spices.
4. Stir in rinsed lentils, vegetable broth, and diced tomatoes with their juices.
5. Bring to a boil, then reduce heat to low, cover, and simmer for 20-25 minutes, or until the lentils are tender.
6. Stir in chopped kale or spinach and cook for an additional 2-3 minutes, or until wilted.
7. Season with salt and pepper to taste.
8. Serve hot with crusty bread for dipping.

Tips:

- You can use any type of lentils for both recipes, but brown lentils tend to hold their shape better.

- Feel free to add other vegetables to the lentil stew, such as potatoes, zucchini, or green beans.

- For a richer flavor, you can add a tablespoon of tomato paste along with the diced tomatoes in the lentil stew recipe.

- You can also add a splash of red wine vinegar or lemon juice to the lentil stew for a touch of acidity.

Chapter 12:

Snack and Appetizer Recipes –

Quick Snacks –

• Shepherd's Pie vs. Turkey Meatloaf: Deciding Between Comfort Food Classics

Both Shepherd's Pie and Turkey Meatloaf are hearty and comforting dishes, perfect for a weeknight meal. Here's a breakdown to help you choose:

Shepherd's Pie:

- **Origin:** Traditionally made with ground lamb (hence the name "Shepherd's"), but ground beef is also common.

- **Components:** A savory layer of seasoned ground meat and vegetables topped with creamy mashed potatoes and baked until golden brown.

- **Flavor Profile:** Rich and savory from the meat and vegetables, balanced by the creamy mashed potatoes.

- **Dietary Considerations:** Not vegetarian or vegan due to the meat content. Can be made gluten-free by using gluten-free breadcrumbs or oats in the filling and ensuring the mashed potatoes are made without wheat flour.

Turkey Meatloaf:

- **Main Ingredient:** Ground turkey, a leaner alternative to ground beef.

- **Preparation:** Similar to a meatball mixture, shaped into a loaf and baked. Often glazed with a sweet and savory sauce.

- **Flavor Profile:** Milder flavor compared to Shepherd's Pie, with the option to customize the glaze for desired sweetness or savory notes.

- **Dietary Considerations:** Can be vegetarian or vegan with plant-based substitutes for the turkey and using a vegan glaze. Gluten-free options are readily available with gluten-free breadcrumbs or oats used as a binder.

Here are some additional factors to consider:

- **Time:** Shepherd's pie requires separate preparation of the meat filling and mashed potatoes, adding a bit more time.

- **Ingredients:** Shepherd's pie requires more ingredients compared to a basic meatloaf recipe.

- **Leftovers:** Both dishes reheat well and are great for meal prepping.

The Verdict:

- **Choose Shepherd's Pie if:** You crave a classic comfort food with a rich and savory flavor profile, and don't mind using ground meat.

- **Choose Turkey Meatloaf if:** You prefer a lighter option with more flexibility in customizing flavors. You also have the option to make it vegetarian or vegan.

– Healthy Appetizers –

• Cucumber Bites with Tuna Salad:

These are light, refreshing, and easy to make, perfect for a summer party or a quick lunch.

Ingredients:

- 1 large cucumber, sliced into 1/2 inch rounds
- 1 (5 oz) can chunk light tuna in water, drained
- 2 tablespoons mayonnaise (or light mayonnaise for a healthier option)
- 1 tablespoon finely chopped red onion
- 1 tablespoon chopped celery
- 1 tablespoon chopped fresh dill (or 1/2 teaspoon dried dill)
- Salt and pepper to taste
- Optional garnishes: dill sprigs, cherry tomatoes (cut in half)

Instructions:

1. Using a melon baller (or spoon), scoop out a small portion of the center from each cucumber slice, creating a little cup.

2. In a bowl, combine drained tuna, mayonnaise, red onion, celery, and dill. Season with salt and pepper to taste.

3. Fill each cucumber cup with the tuna salad mixture.

4. Garnish with a sprig of fresh dill and/or a cherry tomato half (optional).

• Mini Caprese Skewers:

These colorful and flavorful skewers are another easy finger food option. They're perfect for showcasing fresh summer ingredients.

Ingredients:

- Cherry tomatoes
- Mini mozzarella balls (or bocconcini)
- Fresh basil leaves

- Skewers (bamboo or toothpicks)
- Extra virgin olive oil (optional)
- Balsamic glaze (optional)

Instructions:

1. Wash and dry cherry tomatoes and basil leaves.
2. Assemble the skewers by threading a cherry tomato, a mozzarella ball, and a basil leaf onto each skewer, alternating as desired.
3. Drizzle with a touch of olive oil and balsamic glaze for additional flavor (optional).

Tips:

- For the cucumber bites, you can use different herbs in the tuna salad instead of dill, such as parsley or chives.
- If you don't have a melon baller, you can simply use a spoon to create a small indentation in the cucumber slices.
- For the mini Caprese skewers, use grape tomatoes if you don't have cherry tomatoes.

- You can also add a drizzle of pesto sauce to the skewers for extra flavor.

Indulgent Treats –

- Dark Chocolate Bark and Baked Sweet Potato Chips: A Sweet and Salty Treat

Here's a delicious combination for satisfying your sweet and salty cravings:

Dark Chocolate Bark:

This is a simple and customizable treat that requires minimal ingredients and effort.

Ingredients:

- 1 cup chopped dark chocolate (at least 70% cacao for a richer flavor)
- 1/4 cup chopped nuts or seeds (optional)
- 1/4 cup dried fruit (optional)

- 1/4 cup crushed pretzels or rice krispies (optional)

Instructions:

1. Line a baking sheet with parchment paper.

2. In a heatproof bowl, melt the chopped dark chocolate using a double boiler or microwave method (in short bursts, stirring frequently).

3. Once melted and smooth, pour the chocolate onto the prepared baking sheet, spreading it into an even layer.

4. Sprinkle your desired toppings (nuts, seeds, dried fruit, pretzels, or rice krispies) over the melted chocolate.

5. Gently press the toppings into the chocolate to ensure they adhere.

6. Place the baking sheet in the refrigerator for at least 30 minutes, or until the chocolate is completely hardened.

7. Break the bark into pieces and enjoy!

Tips:

- You can use any type of chopped nuts or seeds that you like, such as almonds, walnuts, peanuts, pumpkin seeds, or sunflower seeds.

- Dried fruits like cranberries, cherries, raisins, or chopped apricots add a chewy texture and sweetness.

- Pretzels or rice krispies offer a salty and crunchy contrast to the dark chocolate.

- Get creative with your toppings! You can even drizzle melted white chocolate over the dark chocolate for a marbled effect.

• Baked Sweet Potato Chips:

These healthy and crispy chips are a delicious alternative to regular potato chips. They're naturally sweet and pair well with the dark chocolate bark.

Ingredients:

- 1 large sweet potato

- 1 tablespoon olive oil

- 1/2 teaspoon ground cinnamon (optional)

- 1/4 teaspoon salt
- 1/4 teaspoon black pepper

Instructions:

1. Preheat oven to 375°F (190°C).
2. Wash and dry the sweet potato. Slice the sweet potato very thinly using a sharp knife or mandoline slicer. Aim for even slices for uniform baking.
3. In a large bowl, toss the sweet potato slices with olive oil, cinnamon (if using), salt, and pepper.
4. Arrange the sweet potato slices in a single layer on a baking sheet lined with parchment paper.
5. Bake for 15-20 minutes, or until the edges are golden brown and the chips are crisp.
6. Flip the chips halfway through baking to ensure even browning.
7. Let the chips cool slightly before serving.

Tips:

- For a spicier kick, you can add a pinch of cayenne pepper to the seasoning mix.

- Use a variety of spices to experiment with different flavor profiles.

- Let the sweet potato slices dry completely before baking to ensure they crisp up properly.

- You can also air fry the sweet potato slices instead of baking them.

Chapter 13:

Dessert Recipes –

Light Desserts –

• Yogurt Parfait with Berries:

- **Pros:** Easy to customize with different yogurts, fruits, and toppings. Can be layered for a visually appealing presentation. Great for portion control and meal prepping.

- **Cons:** Requires assembling individual portions. May not be as refreshing as a fruit salad on a hot day.

Fruit Salad:

- **Pros:** Lighter and more refreshing option. Perfect for sharing with a group. Easy to make ahead of time.

- **Cons:** May brown faster than a layered parfait. Less customizable for individual preferences.

Here are some recipe ideas to get you started:

• Yogurt Parfait with Berries:

Ingredients (Serves 1):

- 1 cup plain yogurt (Greek yogurt for added protein)
- 1/2 cup fresh berries (your choice)
- 1/4 cup granola
- 1 tablespoon honey or maple syrup (optional)
- Fresh mint leaves for garnish (optional)

Instructions:

1. In a glass or jar, layer half of the yogurt.
2. Top with half of the berries.
3. Add half of the granola.
4. Repeat layers with remaining yogurt, berries, and granola.
5. Drizzle with honey or maple syrup (optional).
6. Garnish with fresh mint leaves (optional).

Fruit Salad:

Ingredients (Serves 4-6):

- 4 cups mixed fruits (such as berries, melon, grapes, oranges, pineapple)
- 1/4 cup orange juice or lemon juice (optional)
- 2 tablespoons honey or maple syrup (optional)
- Fresh mint leaves for garnish (optional)

Instructions:

1. Wash and chop all fruits into bite-sized pieces.
2. In a large bowl, combine the mixed fruits.
3. Toss with orange juice or lemon juice (optional) to prevent browning.
4. Drizzle with honey or maple syrup (optional) for added sweetness.
5. Garnish with fresh mint leaves (optional).

Tips:

- For the yogurt parfait, you can use flavored yogurt instead of plain yogurt. Just be mindful of added sugar content.

- Chia seeds or chopped nuts can be added to the yogurt parfait for extra texture and nutrients.

- To prevent browning in the fruit salad, toss fruits that brown easily (like apples or bananas) in a little lemon juice or orange juice.

- You can add a splash of liqueur (like Grand Marnier or Amaretto) to the fruit salad for an adult twist (optional).

Baked Goods –

• Banana Bread:

- **Texture:** Dense and moist, cake-like crumb.

- **Flavor:** Sweet and banana-forward, with warm spices like cinnamon and nutmeg often added.

- **Enjoyment:** Typically eaten as a snack or breakfast bread, can be toasted with butter or enjoyed plain.

- **Preparation:** Requires baking in a loaf pan for a set amount of time.

• Oatmeal Cookies:

- **Texture:** Chewy and soft, with a slight crisp on the edges.

- **Flavor:** Varies depending on additional ingredients, but often includes brown sugar, cinnamon, and vanilla. Chocolate chips are a popular addition.

- **Enjoyment:** Typically eaten as a portable snack or dessert.

- **Preparation:** Requires scooping dough balls onto a baking sheet and baking for a shorter time than banana bread.

Here are some factors to consider when choosing:

- **Craving:** If you're looking for something cake-like and substantial, banana bread is a good choice. If you prefer a chewier, bite-sized treat, go for oatmeal cookies.

- **Time:** Oatmeal cookies require less prep time and bake faster than banana bread.

- **Ingredients:** Both require common ingredients, but oatmeal cookies may require rolled oats which banana bread typically doesn't.

Indulgent Desserts –

• Chocolate Avocado Mousse: Rich and Decadent (Vegan!)

This chocolate avocado mousse is a healthy and delicious alternative to traditional mousse. It's surprisingly rich and decadent, and you won't even taste the avocado!

Ingredients (Serves 2):

- 1 ripe avocado, pitted and peeled
- ½ cup raw cacao powder or unsweetened cocoa powder
- ¼ cup maple syrup or honey (or to taste)
- ¼ cup coconut milk (from the top of a can, the thicker cream)
- 1 teaspoon vanilla extract
- Pinch of salt

Instructions:

1. In a blender or food processor, combine the avocado, cacao powder, maple syrup, coconut milk, vanilla extract, and salt.

2. Blend until smooth and creamy, scraping down the sides as needed.

3. Taste and adjust sweetness with additional maple syrup or honey if desired.

4. Divide the mousse between two serving cups or bowls.

5. Chill in the refrigerator for at least 30 minutes, or until set.

6. Enjoy!

Tips:

- For an extra chocolatey flavor, melt 1 ounce of dark chocolate and drizzle it over the top of the mousse before chilling.

- Top your mousse with fresh berries, chopped nuts, or a sprinkle of shredded coconut for added texture and flavor.

- If you don't have coconut milk, you can use another type of milk, but the texture may be slightly thinner.

• Rice Pudding: Creamy Comfort Food

Rice pudding is a classic dessert that's easy to make and endlessly customizable.

Ingredients (Serves 4):

- 1 cup cooked white rice (or brown rice for a more fiber-rich option)
- 2 cups milk (whole milk for a richer pudding, low-fat for a lighter option)
- ¼ cup sugar (or to taste)
- ¼ teaspoon salt
- 1 teaspoon vanilla extract
- 1/2 teaspoon ground cinnamon (optional)
- Nutmeg for garnishing (optional)

Instructions:

1. In a medium saucepan, combine cooked rice, milk, sugar, salt, and vanilla extract.
2. Heat over medium heat, stirring occasionally, until the mixture simmers and begins to thicken.
3. Reduce heat to low and simmer for 15-20 minutes, or until the rice is softened and the pudding reaches your desired consistency. Stir occasionally to prevent sticking.
4. Remove from heat and stir in ground cinnamon (if using).
5. Divide the rice pudding among serving bowls.
6. Let cool slightly before serving.
7. Grate fresh nutmeg over the top of each serving for an extra touch of flavor (optional).

Tips:

- You can add raisins, chopped dried fruit, or chocolate chips to the rice pudding for extra flavor and texture.

- For a richer flavor, whisk in an egg yolk with a tablespoon of milk before adding it to the saucepan in step 2.

- Rice pudding can be served warm, chilled, or at room temperature. Leftovers can be stored in the refrigerator for up to 3 days.

CONCLUSION

We've tasted a lot of different foods during this trip, and each one has added its own melody to the grand symphony of tastes. From the hearty, warming goodness of shepherd's pie to the light, refreshing goodness of cucumber bites with tuna salad, there are so many delicious and healthy foods out there.

Classics like baked salmon with asparagus or lentil stew are always a good choice for people who want a filling and comforting meal. These dishes are great for a cozy night in because they make you feel warm and full. But our taste buds also want to try new things. The bright flavors of stuffed bell peppers or the unexpected richness of chocolate avocado mousse push the limits of what we can do in the kitchen and make new and interesting tastes.

Beauty lies in the freedom to choose. There's a dish out there just waiting to be found, whether you like the ease of banana bread or the versatility of a fruit salad. There are more options than just the recipes. Each step, from choosing fresh herbs and spices to deciding whether to use lean ground turkey in a meatloaf or look into plant-based options, gives us the chance to make it our own, taking into account our own tastes and dietary needs.

Food is more than just sustenance; it's a cultural expression, a social experience, and a form of artistic art. As we explore different cuisines and experiment with ingredients, we connect with customs, celebrate occasions, and express our own culinary identities. The act of cooking itself becomes a form of self-care, a mindful practice that allows us to slow down, enjoy the present moment, and nourish ourselves not just physically, but also emotionally.

The world of food is huge and ever-evolving. New ingredients emerge, cooking methods are refined, and culinary trends affect our palates. This exploration, however, is not meant to be a destination, but rather a delicious trip. Embrace the chance to experiment, to discover new flavors, and to create memories around the table. So, the next time you step into the kitchen, remember the symphony of tastes that awaits. Let your imagination be your guide, and allow yourself to be swept away by the beautiful melody of a well-made meal.